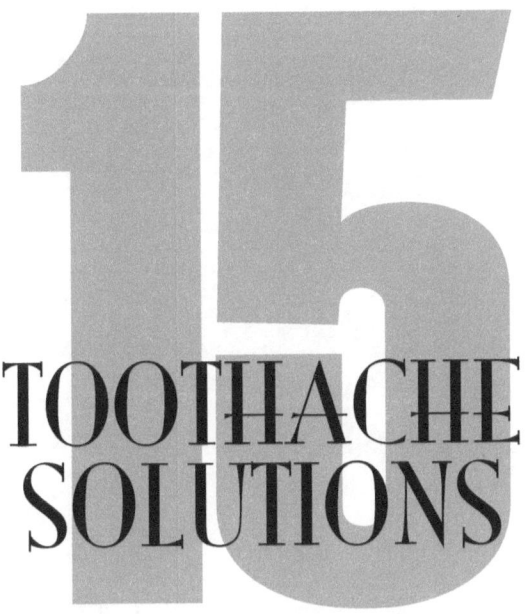

TOOTHACHE SOLUTIONS

DENTAL HEALTH IN YOUR OWN HANDS

BY DR. USHA TANDON, D.D.S.

[THREAD ID: 1-9ATN0E]

United States Copyright Office
[THREAD ID: 1-9AU3AY]
United States Copyright Office

ISBN: 1453710140
ISBN-13: 9781453710142

Library of Congress Control Number: 2011902091

PRAISE FOR *15 TOOTHACHE SOLUTIONS*

In the movie "Peggy Sue Got Married," Peggy Sue asks her grandfather if he could do *anything* different in his past life, what it would be. He thinks a moment and then says, "I would have taken better care of my teeth!"

It gets a small laugh in the movie, but as the years go by, I think Grandpa had the right idea. If only I could go back to my eighteen-year-old self and tell her how to take better care of her teeth.

Better yet, I would hand her Dr. Usha Tandon's book, *15 Toothache Solutions*. It's full of practical information on so many aspects of tooth care. Brushing and flossing are great, but there's a lot more to know if you want to keep your teeth in good shape from your teenage years throughout your life and into your elder years. Finally, *15 Toothache Solutions* gives you ammunition to take charge of your dental health.

If only Grandpa had this book, maybe he could have gotten another wish.

-Georgie Huntington Zaidi

Editor of *Take Charge of Your Diabetes*

THIS BOOK IS DEDICATED TO ALL THE
DENTAL PATIENTS WHO WANT TO
ENJOY GOOD ORAL HEALTH
THROUGHOUT THEIR LIVES.

MY BELIEF AS A DENTIST

Natural human teeth are designed to last as long as we live. It is with our own ignorance and negligence that loss of our teeth happens.

This book will help you overcome the ignorance.

The negligence part is now up to you.

TABLE OF CONTENTS

Food for thought:

Imagine yourself twenty-five and thirty-five years from today and think what kind of appearance, smile, mouth, self confidence, and self esteem you want to have at that time!

INTRODUCTION

AVOID TOOTHACHES, SAVOR YOUR FOOD, AND STAY AWAY FROM DENTURES

Are you worried about painful cavities in your teeth? Do you worry about bleeding and swollen gums? Or, are you simply concerned about teeth that are sensitive and painful to hot and cold foods and drinks?

Whatever your concern may be, it is never too late. The fifteen strategies in this book will steer you in the right direction to solve your toothache problems. After you read this book, you will no longer have to suffer needlessly from tooth pain, discomfort, and premature loss of teeth.

Do You Avoid the Dentist?

Maybe you resist going to the dentist. I remember treating patients with severe dental problems who had never been to a dental office in their lives. It could be because of fear, anxiety, or the high cost of dental treatments. In this short book, I will show you that you have nothing to fear. The fifteen strategies in this book are not only easy to follow, but they will also save you time, discomfort, and expensive repairs.

As a longtime practicing dentist, I realized that patients come to the dentist's office, get their teeth fixed, and then return again and again with different problems. My reason for writing this book is to give you all the information and tools you need to keep your teeth healthy throughout your life. There's no reason to wait—the sooner you put this information and these tools into practice, the sooner you can enjoy the benefits of good health.

Chapter 1

Toothache Solutions—Discover Food Habits that Result in Cavities and Tooth Pain

Do you eat out often? Do you eat fast food? Do you snack on cookies and other processed foods? Or, do you skip breakfast because you are too busy?

Everybody is talking about eating healthy foods these days, as well as what to eat and what not to eat. In this chapter, you will find out not only what foods and food habits hurt your teeth, but also when you should eat your favorite foods. You will also learn what foods you can substitute to create that healthy mouth you want.

How Poor Eating Habits Affect Dental Health

A well-balanced, nutritious diet is the fundamental pillar of good health and well-being. Poor eating habits have a great impact on general health as well as on oral health. You may be so used to eating certain foods or in certain ways that you don't even notice your unhealthy eating habits, which can bring lots of dental problems that result in toothaches.

If you love to eat foods such as cookies, cakes, candies, chocolates, and other soft, sticky foods made of sugar and refined starchy stuff, that could become the biggest culprit for most of your dental problems, as the bacteria in the mouth act on these foods and produce acids. A combination of bacteria and sweet and starchy food, together with acid and saliva, form the dental plaque. This plaque is a sticky coating that collects around the teeth. Acids in the plaque attack enamel, the protective covering on teeth, and cause cavities in teeth. In the beginning, cavities keep progressing slowly without showing any symptoms. By the time you feel pain in the tooth, cavities are already big and gone to deeper layers. If ignored, these can keep expanding and expose the nerve. At this point, you will face severe pain and will need expensive root-canal treatment to save the tooth. Or, the tooth may need to be extracted.

The innocent-looking plaque collected with soft, sticky, and refined foods is also responsible for causing a gum disease called gingivitis. Gingivitis makes the gums get red, tender, and swollen. Teeth can become sensitive and painful if not cared for properly. If gum disease is not treated in time, it can become serious periodontal disease, which is the biggest cause of tooth loss in adults.

Four Poor Eating Habits

1. Are you in the habit of frequent snacking? This is one of those habits that can indirectly result in causing cavities. Why it is not good is because every time you snack, teeth will get exposed to cavity-causing acids for a longer period of time. Repeated attacks of acids break the hard, protective coating of enamel on teeth and result in cavities.

2. Are you one of those people who do not like to eat breakfast in the morning? Skipping meals is another of those bad habits. For example, if you do not eat breakfast or you skip other meals during the day, after a while you may get so hungry that you will grab whatever comes in front of you, and that could be unhealthy, high-calorie junk food responsible for cavities or gum infection.

3. Sports drinks and various kinds of sodas and carbonated soft drinks have adverse effects on teeth by eroding the hard, protective layer of enamel. Thinning of enamel happens, and the layer underneath, called dentin, gets exposed. This results in erosion cavities, which make teeth painful and sensitive. Prolonged exposure of sugar-laden beverages on teeth can also promote dental decay.

4. Eliminating certain foods completely from your diet is not good for general and oral health. Eating variety of foods from all the food groups given to you by the USDA Food Guide Pyramid (United States' Department of Agriculture) will provide you with balanced and healthy nutrition. Healthy food will give you more immunity to fight infections.

A Little Lifestyle Change for a Lot of Happiness

When you decide to create a little lifestyle change and choose moderation in everything, it will go a long way. Eating food with mindfulness, such as not eating on the run or while driving or talking on the phone, and savoring each and every bite will give you long-lasting satisfaction. Stop the habit of skipping meals, especially breakfast, as it is the most important meal of the day. It keeps the metabolism going and gives you energy for the whole day.

For your sweet tooth, eat your favorite foods with meals instead of in between meals. While you are eating meals, saliva is secreted. Saliva, being slightly alkaline, has a protective action that prevents cavities in teeth by neutralizing acids.

Five Foods to Let Go of Now

Stay away from cookies, cakes, candies, chocolates, and other soft, sticky foods. These simple carbohydrates have empty calories and no nutritional value. They have no fiber, and they do not fill you up.

Five Foods to Add

Keep healthy snacks of fresh fruits, like bananas, apples, and papayas, and veg-etables, like celery and carrots, plus nuts easily reachable. Nuts, when eaten in small quantities, are great snacks; walnuts are full of antioxidants and vitamin E, and so are the other nuts. Add avocados in small quanti-ties, because this, too, has the good kind of monounsaturated fat found in nuts and olive oil. Roasted corn on the cob or popcorn without butter can be great snacks.

These complex carbohydrates are plant-based foods and are low in calories. They are high-fiber foods with lot of roughage that take longer to chew, which stimulates the flow of saliva. Saliva washes away the lefto-ver food particles and counteracts mouth acidity.

Seven Tips for Action

1.   Cut down on frequent snacking.

2.   Eat your favorite sweets in moderation and right after your meals rather than in between meals.

3.   Minimize the intake of acidic bever-ages like diet drinks and sport drinks.

4.   Brush twice a day and floss once a day to keep plaque under control. Make a habit to brush your teeth at night as last thing before you go to bed.

5.   Rinse your mouth with water after you eat meals and snacks to remove the leftover food particles.

6.   Plan your menu ahead of time rather than thinking about what to eat when you are hungry.

7.   Rotate your menu to add more variety and interest in preparing healthy foods.

Now that you have learned what foods to eat and when to eat, go to the next chapter to know what to do for your bleeding gums.

Chapter 2

Toothache Solutions—Overcome Gum Disease and Tooth Pain to Regain Happy Teeth

Are you worried about your gums being red, swelling, and bleeding every time you brush your teeth? This is a sign of gum infection called gum disease or gingivitis. At this stage, there is no pain and you might not be aware of it. That is why we call it "silent gum disease." In the beginning, it does not give any sign and symptom, just like high blood pressure, high cholesterol, and so many other medical problems. If not taken care of, it can turn to serious gum disease called periodontal disease. Periodontal disease is responsible for premature loss of teeth in adults.

In this chapter and the next chapter, you will discover why gums get red, swollen, and infected, and how can you stop bleeding from your gums. You will discover how to stay away from advanced stages of periodontal disease, and thus enjoy your natural teeth throughout your life with small easy steps.

Why Does Gum Disease Happen?

Gum disease is one of the most commonly seen diseases in every part of the world. Since it does not give you any sign and symptom in the beginning, it keeps advancing without your knowledge.

1.   Poor oral hygiene is the most important cause for gingivitis. That happens when plaque collects around teeth at gum margins. Plaque is a sticky colorless film of bacteria that constantly forms and sticks around the necks of all the teeth. If soft plaque is not removed daily by proper brushing and flossing, it will keep collecting and will turn to a hard calculus called tartar. Gums get irritated with tartar and become tender and swollen and start bleeding. Infected gums can result in painful teeth.

2.   Hormonal changes in women at puberty, pregnancy, and menopause make them more prone to gingivitis and bleeding gums.

3.   Heredity plays a great role in gum disease, like so many other medical problems. If your parents or grandparents lost their teeth at early age, you are at high risk to face gum problems.

4.   Malnutrition and poor diet play a great role in causing gingivitis. Malnourished people in many other countries suffer

with severe gum disease because of low resistance to infections.

5. Vitamin C is very important for good health of gums. Deficiency of vitamin C can cause bleeding from gums.

6. Stress can indirectly be responsible, as stress undermines your ability to fight infections.

7. Dental fillings that are not done properly, called overhanging fillings, collect plaque and cause infection of gums.

8. Overcrowded teeth are at the biggest risk for gingivitis, as it is difficult to clean and floss them properly to keep them from becoming a source of gum infection.

The Good News for Gum Disease

The best part of gum disease is that it is easily preventable and reversible. It can be prevented with good home care that includes brushing two to three times a day and flossing once a day. Brushing done in a correct manner will remove plaque from all surfaces of teeth. Flossing will remove leftover food particles and plaque from in between teeth where brushes cannot reach.

If soft plaque is not removed, it turns to hard gritty substance called tartar. Tartar cannot be removed by brushing at home. Gum infection can be reversed at this stage with scaling and polishing before it does further damage to deeper tissues and bone around the teeth. Scaling and polishing needs to be done in dental office by a dentist or dental hygienist. With constant care, gums will get to normal health, and you will have a clean mouth like you never had before.

Nine Tips for Action

1. Cut down on unhealthy sugary snacks and processed foods.

2. Brush at night with a soft toothbrush before going to bed.

3. Use antibacterial mouthwash once a day.

4. Rinse your mouth with water after every meal and after sugary snacks.

5. Eat healthy and balanced food with lot of fresh fruits and vegetables. Include oranges, tangerines, and grapefruits, and red and orange bell peppers for extra vitamin C.

6. Be extra cautious and see your dentist more frequently if your parents lost their teeth prematurely and wear dentures.

7.	Consult an orthodontist if your teeth are overcrowded.

8.	Get your teeth restored if you have large overhanging fillings.

9.	Find out why you are stressed out and deal with it patiently.

Are you ready to learn to stop the gum disease from going to an advanced stage of periodontal disease? Then, continue to the next chapter.

Chapter 3

Toothache Solutions—No More Loss of Teeth with Periodontal Disease

Are you getting concerned that your gums bleed a lot and are shrinking or pulling away from your teeth? Are you worried about your loose and painful teeth that give you bad breath? It is a clear signal that your gum disease has gone to the advanced stage called periodontal disease. It is also called chronic destructive periodontitis or pyorrhea. It is with pyorrhea that premature loss of your natural teeth can happen.

In this chapter, you will learn what damage pyorrhea is doing to your teeth and how to stop its progress. You will discover how you can avoid bleeding gums and painful teeth and how you can keep your teeth strong and healthy. You will not want to repeat the same mistakes your parents or grandparents did, if they lost their teeth with pyorrhea and they wear dentures, which are an artificial replacement of teeth. Dentures can be either partial dentures to replace few missing teeth or full dentures to replace all missing teeth.

Why Does Periodontal Disease Happen?

As we talked earlier, gum disease in the beginning is easily preventable and reversible. If it is ignored or left untreated for some time, it keeps progressing below the gums and damages the supporting structures of teeth.

It happens when bacteria from the plaque irritate the gums and start attacking the deeper tissues that attach the gums to the teeth. The gums shrink and pull away from teeth, forming small pockets. With time, pockets become deeper, and ultimately the bacteria starts destroying the bone underneath that supports the teeth. If proper treatment is not started, gums keep bleeding and more bone loss happens, which makes teeth loose and creates spaces in between teeth. Your teeth will become painful and highly sensitive to hot and cold foods. You will smell constant bad odor from your mouth. Your gums will start receding, and roots of teeth will get exposed in the mouth. Roots of teeth are much softer, since they are not covered with a protective layer of enamel, so they decay very easily. Decayed roots are hypersensitive to hot and cold foods and add more discomfort and toothaches.

Why it is Called Chronic Destructive Periodontitis?

It is called chronic destructive periodontitis because the damage done to teeth and its supporting structures becomes permanent damage, which cannot be reversed. If left untreated, your teeth will keep getting loose and ready to fall out. At this stage, it becomes difficult to save the loose teeth, so eventually teeth will have to be pulled out altogether. That is why periodontal disease is the number one cause of loss of teeth in adults and seniors. Periodontal disease causes much more tooth loss than cavities or badly decayed teeth do.

I will never forget that time when my mother lost all her natural teeth at a very young age because of irreversible pyorrhea. She has been wearing a full set of upper and lower dentures since she was forty. In fact, this was the motivating factor for me to become a dentist—so I could help patients and family members to save their precious teeth.

Six Connections Between Periodontal Disease and General Health

Periodontal disease should be paid serious attention. Studies have shown that periodontal disease does not affect your mouth only, but it is also linked with your general health in so many different ways.

1. Healthy gums are essential for a healthy heart. Periodontal disease has shown some connection with cardiovascular disease and stroke. If you have periodontal disease, you are at high risk for heart problems and stroke.

2.   Women suffering with periodontal disease may deliver preterm babies or give birth to underweight babies.

3.   The habit of smoking cigarettes or chewing tobacco puts you at high risk of developing periodontal disease.

4.   Uncontrolled diabetes affects your immune system, and you have less resistance to fight infections, so you are more prone to getting periodontal problems.

5.   Poor nutrition is another factor that contributes to make periodontal disease worse.

6.   Because of your loose teeth or loss of your natural teeth with periodontal disease, you cannot chew your food properly. That will affect your overall health. Loose or missing teeth will affect your smile and speech, also.

Eight Tips for Action

1.   Use your toothbrush as your best tool to maintain your gums' health and, in turn, general health. In addition, use a proxabrush which is a small device that helps remove plaque from wide spaces between teeth which are cre-

ated by recession of gums. Use a floss holder if that seems easier than regular floss. Proxabrush and floss holders are available in drug stores.

2. Get scaling and root planning done in a dental office, as plaque and hard tartar below the gum margins cannot be removed by home care.

3. If you are pregnant, you need to pay attention to early signs of gingivitis and visit your dentist more often to keep your teeth and gums healthy.

4. Stop your smoking habit to cut down your risk for periodontal disease.

5. Keep your diabetes under control.

6. To stop further progress of periodontal disease you must visit the dentist every three months instead of every six months.

7. Follow healthy lifestyle and good eating habits for healthy body and healthy teeth.

8. Eat healthy and nutritious food. Include lots of fresh vegetables and fruits that are full of antioxidants. Deficiency of vitamin C can cause bleeding from gums, so add plenty of fruits from the citrus family.

You have learned how to avoid pain from simple and advanced gum disease. Go to the next chapter if you want to know how to prevent pain from decayed teeth.

Chapter 4

Toothache Solutions—No Need to Suffer from Tooth Pain with Decayed Teeth

Do your teeth hurt every time you eat food, and does your pain get worse with something sweet? Or, do you go through painful experiences with any kind of hot and cold food? It could be because of your decayed teeth. Dental decay is a process that slowly results in destruction of tooth structure, called cavities. It happens with a combination of food and bacteria in your mouth.

In this chapter, you will find out why your teeth get decayed and what you can do to avoid this with ten easy-to-follow steps so you can savor your food without any pain and sensitivity.

What are Cavities?

Cavities are seen as little changes on the surface of teeth caused by bacteria from plaque. Dental plaque is sticky, colorless film formed on teeth because of bad oral hygiene. Cavities do not give pain or any other symptom in the beginning. Then the changes in teeth keep getting bigger, and cavities look like tiny holes as decay gets in deeper layers of teeth. That is when sensitivity and pain starts with hot and cold food. If not treated, cavities get closer to the nerve—called pulp—that gets infected and gives severe pain. This is the time when you either have to face tooth loss or need expensive root canal treatment to save your tooth.

What are Most Common Places for Cavities?

Molars and premolars are the most common places for cavities. Why? Because chewing surfaces of these teeth have lots of pits and grooves that are difficult to keep clean. So, those are easy places for bacteria to sit and hide.

Another common place to get cavities is between the teeth on areas called interproximal surfaces. These are the areas where a tooth contacts the adjacent tooth. As these areas are difficult to reach with a toothbrush, only dental floss or other flossing devices can remove plaque from these surfaces of teeth. If flossing is not done properly, plaque will keep collecting in between teeth and cause painful cavities.

Roots of teeth are highly prone to get cavities if they are exposed in the mouth because of gum recession. Exposed roots collect lots of plaque and are easy targets for root decay. Why? Because roots of teeth are not covered with a hard layer of enamel on them, they are much softer than crowns of teeth.

What Makes Cavities on Teeth?

1. Dental cavities are the result of poor oral hygiene that shows up as plaque around the teeth. Plaque is a sticky, colorless film of bacteria that keeps building continuously on your teeth day and night. This innocent-looking bacterial film is the major culprit for causing most dental diseases, including cavities in teeth.

2. Cavities are formed when you eat lots of soft, sweet, and starchy foods. The bacteria from the plaque use the sweet stuff to produce acid that attacks the enamel on the teeth. With repeated attacks of acid, the protective and hard layer of enamel finally breaks down. That results in making small to big holes in teeth called cavities.

3. Your frequent snacking can be the cause of your cavities. The more often you eat, the more often bacteria feed on these foods and produce acids that attack teeth and lead to cavities.

4.   Whenever you have dry mouth, your chances of getting cavities keep increasing. With dry mouth, you have less saliva in your mouth. Saliva, being slightly alkaline in nature, has a protective action in counteracting the acids produced by bacteria in mouth plaque. In this process, saliva protects the teeth from cavities. Anything that causes dry mouth can result in cavities. For example, if you sleep with an open mouth, your mouth will get dry and make you more prone to cavities.

5.   When roots of your teeth get exposed in your mouth because of gum disease, you are likely to get cavities on root surfaces. As roots of teeth are difficult to keep clean, they get covered with plaque very quickly.

Proper Method for Brushing

Place a soft-bristle toothbrush at the junction of gums and teeth, tip the brush slightly toward the gum line, and brush gently with short back-and-forth movements without putting too much pressure on the toothbrush. Too much force never helps clean teeth better. In fact, it damages teeth and pushes the gums away. Start at one end of the jaw and move the brush slowly to the other end. Brushing strokes should always overlap each other. Brush only few teeth at a time. Start from chewing surfaces of back teeth, where bacteria are more likely to hide in grooves and fissures. Then brush the outside surfaces toward the cheek side and end on inside surfaces toward the tongue side of all teeth. Then try to brush the back surfaces of the last teeth in the mouth.

Always brush gently for at least two to three minutes. Replace your toothbrush after every four to five months or even earlier if the bristles seem damaged. Make sure that you wash your brush after using and keep it in sunny place where it can dry before the next use. Do not keep the brush in a cover, as wet brushes will harbor bacteria. To prevent cross-contamination, never share your toothbrush with anybody else. Electric toothbrushes are good and are easier to use than manual toothbrushes. They do good job in cleaning the teeth if used properly. They are a great help for people with arthritis or with muscle weakness in their hands.

Proper Method for Flossing

Use floss to remove plaque from in between teeth, called interdental areas, where toothbrushes cannot reach. Flossing will be effective only if done in a correct manner. Take sixteen to eighteen inches of dental floss. Wrap the floss around your middle fingers, leaving about two inches of floss in between to work with. With gentle movements, try to scrape the side of each tooth a few times by back-and-forth motion without injuring the gum tissue between the two teeth. In the end, try to floss the back side of the last teeth in your dental arch also.

Ten Tips for Action

1.   Remember to brush your teeth at night before going to bed and not to eat anything after that. In addition, brush once or twice during the day.

2.   Floss your teeth at least once a day.

3.   Rinse your mouth with plain water after every time you eat and snack.

4.   Cut down on unhealthy, soft, sticky, and sweet foods.

5.   Cut down on snacking in between meals.

6.   Make sure that you do not sleep with your mouth open. Always breathe through your nose so you do not get dry mouth.

7.   Do not ignore the first sign of pain and sensitivity in your teeth.

8.   Use oral rinse with fluoride every day that has the ADA (American Dental Association) seal of approval.

9.   Use fluoride toothpaste, as fluoride helps to strengthen the teeth.

10. Get routine dental cleanings and check-ups twice a year. A dentist can pinpoint the cavities at their starting point and save your teeth before further damage is done.

You have learned how to avoid cavities and pain in teeth. If you want to know why untreated cavities can cause dental abscesses and root-canal infection, then go to next chapter.

Chapter 5

Toothache Solutions—No Need to Worry About Dental Abscesses and Infected Root Canals

Have you ever felt the kind of severe tooth pain, tenderness, and swelling around the tooth that does not let you sleep at night? Or your tooth is so hypersensitive to hot and cold that you cannot eat your food properly? These symptoms could be indicative of severe infection of root canal and dental abscess.

In this chapter, you will get to know the sequence of causes that result in a severely infected tooth. You will learn how to avoid extreme pain and discomfort with a few precautions taken earlier so you can sleep through the night without tooth pain and savor your food with no sensitivity in teeth.

What is Root Canal Infection and Why Does it Happen?

It starts as a small, simple cavity in the tooth. The cavity, in the beginning, is painless. This is the time when only a dentist can discover the cavity and fix it easily. If ignored, the cavity will keep getting bigger and deeper. Finally, it reaches the middle part of the tooth, where it irritates and infects the pulp. The pulp is a soft tissue protected inside the center of hard shell of tooth. Most people call it the nerve, which makes it easier to understand. Infection damages the nerve and eventually makes the nerve die. That can result in extreme pain, swelling, and abscess around the tooth. Some patients describe it as one of the most painful experiences. Many female patients call it very similar to labor pain! This excruciating pain is the result of severe decay in the tooth.

Infection of pulp can also happen with broken large fillings or cracked teeth which irritate the pulp and cause sensitivity to hot and cold foods and beverages. You will have difficulty eating and chewing food. If it is your front tooth, you will feel pain while biting on hard or raw foods. Pain will get worse with little touch or pressure on the tooth.

Any trauma or injury to the tooth or a severe blow to your face can cause infection of pulp. Sometimes, your tooth may have no symptoms initially, but the color of your tooth may change from light yellow to dark brown gradually. That happens when your tooth gets exposed to low-grade infection, but for a longer time, called chronic infection. It indicates that the nerve has died slowly and will need root canal treatment to save the tooth.

What is Root Canal Treatment?

Root canal treatment is also called RCT for short. It is a dental procedure to save your tooth when the nerve in the tooth is infected and is partially or fully dead. The nerve or pulp is removed, and the tooth is filled with a special filling material so it can function like a normal tooth. Later, a permanent restoration, such as porcelain crown, is placed on this tooth.

What is the Purpose of Root Canal Treatment?

If the infected tooth is not treated quickly, it can develop an abscess at the tip of the root inside the bone. An abscess is like a little pocket of pus. In severe cases, a patient may get excruciating pain, swelling of the jaw, fever, and other uncomfortable feelings.

The purpose of the root canal treatment is to fix the damage done by severe decay and save the tooth from extraction. The dentist who specializes in this field is called an endodontist, though some general dentists can do RCT as well.

Save the Tooth with RCT or Extract It?

In old times, people used to get their teeth pulled out under these circumstances. Even at present times, many patients want to get the tooth pulled out rather than save it with RCT. The main reason I have found was their fear, based on horror stories they had heard from other people, that RCT is extremely painful, takes too many visits to dental office, or costs too much money. With new technology, RCT is very easy and safe and is done in one or two dental visits.

Your root-canal-treated tooth can become fragile and brittle, since it had a deep cavity or a large filling, or it was a broken tooth to start with. So, after the completion of the treatment, get the proper restoration of a ceramic or gold crown placed on the tooth. After that, your tooth will function as a normal healthy tooth for all practical purposes and will last for years to come.

On the other hand, if you get your tooth pulled out instead, you will have a missing tooth in your mouth. A missing tooth will lead to bite problems, such as when neighboring teeth and opposing teeth start shifting to fill the gap, and will lead to many other bite-related complications. You can get a missing tooth replaced with an implant, fixed crown and bridge work, or partial denture, but remember, nothing is like your own natural tooth.

Six Tips for Action

Many of my patients ask me this question: "How can I avoid root canal infection?" Let me share the answer with you.

1. Get your teeth fixed at the first sign of decay and thus prevent the painful situation. Do not ignore the symptoms of cavities in your teeth, such as a dull pain in the tooth, sensitivity to hot and cold, or a tiny hole in the tooth.

2. Pay attention if food is getting impacted in between your teeth and you feel like removing the leftover food with a toothpick. This is another signal of a cavity on the surface of your tooth that is next to adjacent tooth, which is called a proximal cavity.

3. Schedule routine check-ups in your dental office. A dentist can notice decay forming at the very initial stage by probing and with dental X-rays. Small cavities need a simple filling to fix and save your tooth at that time, with minimum discomfort and little cost.

4. Wear a mouth guard while playing sports, and save your teeth from trauma or a blow to the face.

5. Don't wait too long to get broken fillings or cracked teeth fixed.

6. Pay attention if your teeth get sensitive or you feel pain while eating. Let your dentist check it.

When you take care of these symptoms, the sudden, severe pain will not happen.

Now you know how to save your teeth from root canal infection, go to the next chapter to know what to do for painful wisdom teeth.

Chapter 6

Toothache Solutions—Dealing with Painful Wisdom Teeth: Extract Them or Keep Them

Is the pain in back of your mouth not letting you sleep? Is your jaw tender or swollen? Maybe eating and swallowing food is painful for you?

You are not alone. Your wisdom teeth are probably coming in. We all have gone through this experience. Wisdom teeth are known to cause pain every time they erupt in the mouth because they are either partially or fully impacted in most cases.

In this chapter, you will understand why wisdom teeth bring so much pain and discomfort. You will discover how to deal with them and whether your wisdom teeth need to be extracted or not.

Why They Are Called Wisdom Teeth?

Wisdom teeth are the last four molars that spring forth at the farthest place in the back of your mouth, one in each corner. Their name comes from the idea that they come in at a later age, around adulthood, from eighteen to twenty-two, when we are supposed to be much wiser and more responsible. When they come in, you will have a full set of thirty-two teeth in your mouth. They are often called third molars.

Why Do Wisdom Teeth Get Impacted?

When teeth are not able to erupt in the mouth through the gum tissue and bone, they are called impacted. As wisdom teeth are the last molars to come in the mouth, they are not left with enough space to accommodate them because of the twenty-eight teeth already present there. So, your wisdom teeth may not come out fully in proper position in the dental arch.

You may get wisdom teeth partially impacted when only part of the tooth is visible in the mouth. Or, your tooth may be completely impacted in your jaw. This means it may stay totally under the gum tissue and bone. It is possible that your wisdom teeth may fully erupt in your mouth, but they may be either crooked or angled toward the roots of neighboring teeth because of lesser space.

Disadvantages of Impacted Wisdom Teeth

Wisdom teeth act as a source of infection in the mouth, and they can damage the other teeth in many different ways.

In partially impacted wisdom teeth, only part of the tooth is visible in the mouth and the rest is hidden within the flap of gums. Leftover food particles, plaque, and bacteria collect around them and inside the flap. It becomes extremely difficult to brush and keep that area clean. This results in gum infection, abscesses, and swelling around the wisdom teeth, causing constant pain. You will notice bad breath and a bad taste in your mouth. In severe cases, you may get swelling of the jaw and face, and difficulty in eating and swallowing food. It may become difficult for you to open your mouth wide; this is called trismus.

Your crooked wisdom teeth collect lots of plaque and are likely to get painful cavities between the teeth, called proximal cavities. It may be extremely difficult for you to keep the crooked teeth clean and floss properly.

Your misaligned wisdom teeth can slowly push your other permanent molars in front of them, resulting in crowding of teeth. That can change the whole bite, leading to more complications.

Your wisdom teeth that are angled toward the teeth in front of them can do lot of damage to adjacent teeth and the bone supporting those teeth. That can result in serious gum disease and other related problems.

Should I Keep Wisdom Teeth or Extract Them?

There are two points of view to consider.

As your wisdom teeth are so far back, your toothbrush may not reach there to keep them clean and free of plaque. So, they may harbor bacteria inside the mouth. Results include severe pain, consistent bad breath, and swelling around the tooth. With my own partially impacted wisdom teeth, I remember facing so much pain, recurrent infection, and restricted ability to open my mouth. Once I got them extracted, it was a big relief. After that, it became much easier to maintain good oral hygiene.

On the other hand, however, though quite uncommon, wisdom teeth can be a big asset, and you may want to keep them if they are symptomless and are in proper position in the dental arch.

Seven Tips for Action

1. Gargle with salt and warm water a few times a day to reduce the pain.

2. Eat soft food, and eat in smaller bites.

3. Do not open your mouth too wide.

4. Brush gently with a soft toothbrush to remove trapped food and debris.

5. Check with your dentist if you need antibiotics.

6. Get an oral exam and X-rays from your dentist to see if a tooth needs to be extracted.

7. Check with oral and maxillofacial surgeons—specialists for surgical procedures.

Now that you have learned how to take care of painful wisdom teeth, go to the next chapter to know which oral habits are damaging your teeth.

Chapter 7

Toothache Solutions—Discover Bad Oral Habits that Damage the Teeth and Result in Tooth Pain

Are you one of those who love to chew on ice cubes and end up with broken or chipped teeth? Or maybe you bite on hard nut shells and break your old fillings and crowns? Maybe you are like my husband, who used to take great pride for his strong teeth. He tried to open every bottle with his teeth, and he ended up with sensitive teeth and chipped corners of teeth before he stopped that habit.

In this chapter, you will get to know so many other bad oral habits that can damage your teeth and result in pain and sensitivity. Once you learn the basic purpose of teeth, you will not have to suffer with unnecessary tooth-ache problems.

Do You Have Any of These Six Bad Oral Habits?

1. Bad oral habits are unhealthy and damage your teeth when you use your teeth for other purposes than

eating, chewing and cutting foods for which they were meant for.

2.   Using your teeth as a cutting tool to tear packaging materials will most likely break your old fillings or crack your teeth.

3.   You can break your teeth if you have habit of biting on hard nut shells such as walnuts, almonds, or pistachios. I see this often with some of my family members. One patient had the bad habit of chewing on pencils. Every pencil sitting on his desk was chewed up. Chewing pencils may also damage your teeth. A few friends complained of sensitivity and pain because of broken and chipped corners of teeth when they tried to bite and peel the hard skin of fresh sugarcane.

4.   You will get small divots in your teeth if you like to hold objects with teeth, like needles and paper clips. This is not a good habit as it makes the edges of teeth rough and sharp, which can break easily and make teeth sensitive and painful. I remember seeing a patient, when I was a dental student in India, with small divots in his front teeth. He told me he is a tailor and holds needles with his teeth while sewing clothes.

5.   Some bad oral habits are signs of nervousness. For example, the habits

of clenching teeth and night grinding could be indications of stress and tension. The same is true for nail biting and cheek biting. These are commonly seen in teenage children, though they can happen at any age. You may bite your nails when you are nervous or bored. Lip biting is another bad habit.

6. Some dental patients have another bad oral habit that they are not aware of. For example, eating with one side of your mouth only is called unilateral mastication and is not considered a healthy habit, either. In fact, it is very damaging, as overuse of one side and underuse of the other will cause imbalance of chewing forces. This can happen if you have missing teeth or painful teeth in one side of your mouth and you avoid eating food on that side. Eating food is an exercise for teeth and has to be done on both sides equally.

Why These Habits are Bad

First of all, biting on hard objects can chip, break, or crack your teeth at a wrong angle. Teeth can become sensitive to hot and cold temperatures. Edges of teeth become rough and sharp, and can break easily.

Depending upon where the fracture line is, your tooth can cause you sharp, shooting pain. Old fillings and porcelain crowns can break. Not only do you face discomfort and pain, but you will also need expensive treatments to replace all fillings and crowns.

A cheek-biting habit can cause ulceration on the inner lining of cheeks and hurts with hot and spicy food. A nail-biting habit can cause oral infections if nails are not kept clean all the time. Not only do nails look ugly, but teeth can get chipped or may get fracture lines and get worn down. Lip biting can result in painful ulceration on lips that may get infected and cause pain.

Eight Tips for Action

1.   Remind yourself that teeth are meant for eating and cutting food only. So, resist the habit of using your teeth for opening lids and biting on any hard object other than food.

2.   Decrease the visibility and accessibility of needles, paper clips, and pencils until you get over this habit.

3.   Keep your nails trimmed all the time. Find the underlying cause of nervousness if you bite your nails or clench your teeth because of that. Take few deep breaths when you are angry or stressed out. Take some classes of gentle stretches of yoga and medita-

tion that help to calm the mind and heal through relaxation.

4. Get chipped and broken teeth fixed before further damage is done.

5. Get sharp and rough edges smoothened in your dental office before they break at the wrong angle and cause severe pain.

6. Make a commitment to quit the habit of biting your lips, cheeks, and nails.

7. Get broken fillings and crowns restored and replaced before they start hurting you badly.

8. Make it a habit to eat food equally on both sides of your mouth. If you have decayed teeth or missing teeth that don't let you eat equally, get them restored and replaced before severe problems can happen.

Now that you have learned to resist bad oral habits, go to the next chapter to learn how women can go through pregnancy with the least worry of tooth pain.

Chapter 8

Toothache Solutions—No Need to Worry About Tooth Pain in Pregnant Women

Are you surprised that your gums are red and bleed easily now that you are pregnant? Do you worry about what to do if your teeth start hurting during pregnancy?

In this chapter, you will discover why these toothache problems happen. You will know why you have to be careful when you choose your antibiotics. You will learn which foods to avoid and nine tips to help you to go through pregnancy worry-free.

Why Do Gums Get Red and Puffy in Pregnancy?

As a woman, you face hormonal changes at so many stages in your life, such as puberty, pregnancy, and menopause. Any time there is a hormonal change in your body, it affects the health of your gums. So, pregnancy makes you more vulnerable to getting red, puffy, and swollen gums that bleed easily. This is called "pregnancy gingivitis." It is because of the inflammation of the gums caused by bacteria in the plaque. The high levels of hormones could be partially respon- sible for it. If you don't take care of gingivi- tis in time, it can turn to an advanced stage of gum disease called periodontal disease. In periodontal disease, infection goes to deeper tissues that support the teeth. That can result in swollen, tender, and painful gums. You may also get bad breath.

What is the Effect of Gum Disease on New-born Babies?

Gum disease is not good for the developing baby. If you have been suffering with peri- odontal disease, you are at high risk of deliv- ering a premature baby. Or, your baby may be born too small, with low birth weight.

Why Do Women Get More Cavities in Preg-nancy?

Cavities are formed when sweet, starchy food remains around the teeth. The bacteria from the plaque use the sweet stuff to pro- duce acid that attacks the enamel on the teeth. Hormonal change exaggerates the effect of acids in plaque, and this makes you more vulnerable to get decay in your teeth. On top of that, you are likely to eat food at short intervals in pregnancy and snack fre- quently. That may add more cavities in teeth because the more often you eat, the more your teeth will get exposed to cavity-causing acids.

Which Foods to Avoid and Which Foods to Eat?

Avoid candies, cookies, and sweet and starchy foods with empty calories. Stay away from high-calorie junk foods, processed foods, and artificial sweeteners.

Replace them with healthy snacks such as fresh fruits, low fat yogurt, and nuts—but in moderation. Almonds are a great snack, as they have good monounsaturated fat, just like avocados. Fill up on high-fiber foods like whole grains, lentils, legumes, and beans. Add lots of vegetables to your daily diet and extra helpings of low-fat dairy products.

Which Antibiotics are Harmful and Should Be Avoided?

Because babies' teeth start forming before they are born, there is an antibiotic that you need to avoid during pregnancy, called tetracycline. Tetracycline is a drug known to cause very dark stains on your baby's teeth if you take it while you are pregnant. These are called internal stains, the kind of stains that will not go away with polishing and bleaching. The good news is that once the teeth are fully formed, tetracycline does not do any harm.

Nine Tips for Action

1.   For a healthy baby, keep your gums in good condition. Brush your teeth two or three times a day and floss once a day—at least—to keep plaque under control and to avoid gingivitis.

2.   Inform your dentist if you are pregnant.

3.   Avoid taking the antibiotic tetracycline, or replace it with a different antibiotic.

4.   Cut down on snacking in between meals.

5.   Get your routine cleaning and regular check-ups done earlier than six months during pregnancy if you have signs of gum disease.

6.   To avoid cavities, rinse your mouth with plain water after every meal and after snacking to remove leftover food particles.

7.   Take calcium supplements to help grow healthy babies with stronger teeth.

8.   Eat a healthy and balanced diet.

9.   Add vitamin D supplement, as it is essential for absorption of calcium in the body.

Go to the next chapter to learn how much damage night grinding could be doing to your teeth.

Chapter 9

Toothache Solutions—Get Rid of Mouth Pain Caused by Night Grinding and Teeth Clenching

A re you wondering why your mouth feels tired or sore when you wake up in the morning? You might not be aware that you are grinding your teeth during sleep. This habit of clenching and grinding of teeth is called bruxism. This could be a signal of some serious underlying problem.

In this chapter, you will find out what could be the underlying cause for your clenching and grinding habit and what damage it is doing to your teeth. Once you learn how to stop this habit, you will save yourself from so much pain and discomfort.

What Makes You Grind Your Teeth?

Under normal conditions, upper and lower teeth are supposed to meet in a definite arrangement called normal occlusion or normal bite. Bruxism can happen when your teeth are not aligned correctly. It means when you close your mouth, your upper and lower teeth meet with each other in an abnormal bite called malocclusion. The reason for your malocclusion could be overcrowding of teeth. That can happen with early loss of your natural teeth causing empty space between teeth. The surrounding teeth and opposing teeth start to drift out to fill that space and change your bite. Overcrowding can also happen with discrepancy in size of jaw and teeth. A smaller-sized jaw cannot accommodate big teeth, resulting in overcrowding of teeth. This could potentially lead to cavities in teeth, gum disease and pain in jaws.

Sometimes you grind your teeth because of certain stresses and strains of life. It is possible that you clench your teeth when you are nervous or under a lot of pressure or tension. In my dental practice, I saw some children who were grinding their teeth while sleeping around the time of their final exams.

I have met people who are not in the habit of night grinding, but they keep clenching their teeth when they are extremely angry.

Two Forms of Night Grinding or Teeth Clenching

Night grinding can be very mild or infrequent, and you may not be aware of it. Usually, either your spouse will notice it, or the person sleeping next to you will complain about it. In case of children, it is the parents who usually point out the problem. This kind of night grinding does not do much damage to teeth or jaws, and you might outgrow it.

In severe night grinding, your teeth can get flat and worn down. Your old fillings can get chipped and cracked. You can wake up with a headache and tired facial muscles. Your teeth will get sensitive and painful. It could be very damaging to your teeth and facial structures. I know some patients who felt pain radiating to their ears and faced problems in the temporomandibular joint. This is the joint that connects the lower jaw with the upper jaw in front of the ears and helps in opening and closing the mouth. It is called TMJ for short.

Eight Tips for Action

1. Learn to deal with stressful situations, and keep yourself calm if stress is the cause. Include some relaxation techniques in your daily routine. Simple and mild stretches of yoga with deep breathing can be very helpful. Yoga seems physical in nature, but it is great for balancing the mind-body-spirit connection. Yoga done with meditation reduces stress and brings calmness and makes you a happier person.

2. Exercise regularly. Exercise is important as it releases some mood-elevating hormones called endorphins.

3. Consult your dentist or physician if you require psychological help to deal with underlying issues of stress.

4. Consult an orthodontist about over-crowding of teeth, uneven teeth, or extra space between teeth. An ortho-dontist is the specialist who straightens the teeth into proper alignment.

5. Get a custom-made night guard or mouth guard to protect your teeth from grinding. Wear it at night while sleeping. This will help by cushioning the teeth and by separating the upper teeth from the lower teeth.

6. Get your old broken fillings restored.

7. Get your fractured and cracked teeth fixed before further damage is done.

8. Replace your missing teeth to avoid future overcrowding and related complications.

Go to the next chapter to know how much damage smoking can do to your whole mouth.

Chapter 10

Toothache Solutions—Understand How Cigarette Smoking is Hurting your Mouth

Do you notice the change in your looks and smile that smoking has caused? Do you dislike your stained and rotten teeth? Maybe you are embarrassed about your smoker's breath? Are you worried about what your smoking habit is doing to the health of your mouth, teeth, and gums?

You probably always knew that cigarette smoking is not good for your overall health and puts you at high risk for lung cancer. But what you may not have known is that smoking is a risk factor for oral cancer as well. In this chapter, you will learn how to take care of your discolored teeth and gum disease and how to avoid losing your natural teeth. You will get to know the early symptoms of oral cancer, which could be life saving.

"What You Know Now, You Can Never Not Know Again"

Cigarettes and chewing tobacco are damaging to the health of your mouth, teeth, gums, and body.

Any kind of smoking—whether it is cigarette, pipe, or cigar smoking—and simply tobacco chewing all raise the risk of developing oral cancer. Oral cancer can happen anywhere in the mouth, including any part of the tongue, the inner lining of the cheeks and lips, the roof and floor of the mouth, the throat, and the gums. If not diagnosed and treated at its earliest stage, oral cancers can be disfiguring and life threatening.

Smoking and Gum Disease Are Connected

If you smoke consistently, you are also at high risk for gum disease. Nicotine is a toxic substance in tobacco that damages your gums. That makes you more prone to collect plaque and the hard tartar called calculus. Once calculus is accumulated on teeth, you cannot remove it with your home care. Your gums will recede underneath the calculus, and your roots will become exposed. Since roots are not covered with a hard, protective layer of enamel, they are soft and decay very easily. Exposed roots cause sensitivity to hot and cold foods, and brushing the teeth becomes very uncomfortable. Simple gum disease, if not treated in time, can cause deep pockets and ultimately loss of bone and tissues that support your teeth, resulting in premature loss of many of your teeth.

Smoking and the Healing Process

In addition, because of smoking, the healing process is delayed after surgical procedures. If you smoke, you will face the problem of delayed healing after extraction of teeth or any other dental procedure.

Smoking and Dry Mouth

With smoking, there is reduction in the flow of saliva in your mouth, which leads to dry mouth. Saliva keeps the mouth wet and washes away leftover food particles. With less saliva, food particles cling to the teeth and begin the decay process, leading to cavities and related pain and discomfort. Dry mouth is responsible for a typical kind of unpleasant odor called smoker's breath. If you smoke consistently, your sense of taste and smell are reduced also.

Smoking and Discolored Teeth

Tobacco chewing and smoking cause dark yellow or brown stains on teeth and the tongue, which are visible from a distance. These dark stains on teeth are very stubborn stains and usually are difficult to remove with normal brushing at home and with routine cleaning and polishing in a dental office. You will need a tooth whitening or bleaching procedure done by a dentist to give your teeth a normal, sparkling look.

Smokeless Tobacco

Smokeless tobacco has an additional disadvantage. With smokeless tobacco, you are more prone to get cavities and related pain and discomfort in teeth, as it contains sugar.

Eight Tips for Action

1. Make a commitment to quit your tobacco habit, whether it is cigarette, cigar, or pipe smoking, or smokeless tobacco. Quitting is the most important step for your general and oral health.

2. Keep regular visits to your dental office for precancerous screening, since early detection and treatment is life saving.

3. Get scaling, polishing, and root planning done in your dental office to keep your gums healthy and to avoid any future tooth loss.

4.   Get decayed roots and other cavities fixed before they get bigger and start hurting.

5.   Use fluoride gel or fluoride mouthwash to strengthen exposed roots.

6.   Pay attention to any ulcers or white and red patches in your mouth. Contact your dentist if you find any.

7.   Consult a cosmetic dentist to bleach or place veneers on your teeth for heavy stains that don't go away with scaling and polishing.

8.   Avoid secondhand smoke, which is equally dangerous.

Now that you have digested this information, are you ready to go to the next chapter to learn how to avoid sensitivity in teeth and enjoy your favorite foods?

Chapter 11

Toothache Solutions—No More Sensitive Teeth: Enjoy Your Coffee and Ice Cream

Are you scared of taking your first sip of hot tea or coffee because your teeth are sensitive? Do you resist your favorite ice cream, cold water, or hot soup because you fear the shooting pain in your teeth?

In this chapter, you will discover what makes your teeth sensitive. You will learn easy-to-follow tips to avoid all those causes so you can enjoy your food without any fear of pain or discomfort.

What Does Sensitivity Mean in Regard to Teeth?

Sensitivity can be described as a painful response or discomfort in one tooth or in all the teeth. It starts with a sharp, shooting pain every time you eat hot or cold, sweet or sour, or spicy foods. Sometimes a cold blast of air can hurt. Many of my patients complain that even brushing their teeth became difficult with sensitive teeth, as that would hurt them, too.

Eight Causes That Make Your Teeth Sensitive

1. Poor oral hygiene and a lot of plaque build-up around your teeth. Plaque is a thin film of bacteria that produces cavities in the teeth near the gum margin. These cavities make teeth painful and sensitive.

2. Receding gums and exposed roots of your teeth because of gum disease or aging. Exposed roots are sensitive to hot, cold, sweet, and sour foods. Roots are not covered with a hard and protective layer of enamel and thus are susceptible to root decay that makes teeth very painful.

3. Brushing your teeth with a hard toothbrush or brushing too vigorously. Both habits can damage the protective layer of enamel. Your gums get pushed away, and roots of teeth get exposed in the mouth. This condition is called Stillman's clefts, and it forms along the gum margin. These exposed areas cause extreme sensitivity to hot and cold. Even normal eating and drinking can become uncomfortable. Breathing in cold air can hurt.

4. When teeth are not brushed or flossed properly, they collect plaque and tartar around them and start gum infection called gingivitis. Gums get red and swollen and bleed easily. Infected gums make teeth sensitive and painful.

5. Clenching or grinding your teeth at night. Night grinding could be related to a stressful situation, tension, or anxiety. Teeth enamel wears off and causes erosion cavities that are responsible for sensitive teeth.

6. Repeated exposure of teeth to acidic foods, such as sour pickles and chutneys, lemons, or diet drinks and sport drinks, makes the enamel wear off. If drinks are consumed slowly, it is even worse because of the extra time the teeth are exposed to acids. This is one of the biggest causes for sensitivity in teeth. Generally, people think that soft drinks are unhealthy because of their sugar content. In fact, the acidic effect is much more harmful.

7. Your broken fillings and crowns or chipped and cracked teeth can be responsible for sensitivity. Severity of pain and sensitivity depends upon the where the break point is.

8. Sensitive teeth could be related to thinning of enamel on your teeth, called erosion cavities. Such cavities

indicate that you may be suffering from acid reflux from the stomach, either with gastroesophageal reflux disease (GERD) or with bulimia nervosa. The acids from your stomach come into the mouth and start eroding tooth enamel.

Eleven Tips for Action

1. Do not put too much pressure on your toothbrush because brushing with force does not help clean better. Brush softly and gently.

2. Start using an electronic toothbrush, as it has controlled pressure and cleans well.

3. Minimize your consumption of soft drinks. Try to finish them in a shorter time.

4. Practice meticulous plaque control with proper methods of brushing at home and regular cleaning in your dental office to avoid cavities, root decay, and gum infection.

5. Use desensitizing toothpaste meant for sensitive teeth.

6. Use fluoride gel or mouth rinse as recommended by your dentist.

7.   Eat foods that are at room temperature. Avoid extreme hot or cold drinks until sensitivity is gone.

8.   Go easy on spices, sour pickles, and cilantro and tamarind chutneys until sensitivity is gone.

9.   Use some relaxation techniques if you are grinding your teeth because of stress or tension. You may also need a night guard to stop grinding.

10.   Get your broken teeth or fillings fixed before they get worse.

11.   Consult your physician if you are suffering from GERD or bulimia.

Go to the next chapter to recognize the life-threatening signs of oral cancer.

Chapter 12

Toothache Solutions—Recognize the Early Signs of Oral Cancer and Related Mouth Pain

Are you concerned about having difficulty in chewing or swallowing food? Do you have trouble moving your tongue around in your mouth? Do you worry about canker sores or white and red patches in your mouth that do not heal?

In this chapter, you will discover how to recognize symptoms of precancerous lesions, because lesions are painless in the beginning. If not treated in time, they can become life threatening. This chapter will explain how dental screenings could be life saving. When diagnosed early, oral cancers can be completely curable.

Eight Oral Symptoms to Watch Out For

Just like most of the cancers in the body, oral cancers can be painless and symptomless in the early stages. They can start at any place in the mouth, including lips, tongue, gums, palate, floor of mouth, or inner lining of cheeks. The following are some signs to watch for:

1. Any kind of ulcers and canker sores that do not heal for about two weeks.

2. Redness on the mucosal lining of mouth or for red patches on the tongue.

3. Thick and velvety white or gray patches, which are commonly seen at the side of the tongue or on the inner lining of the cheeks. This is called leukoplakia.

4. Unexplained numbness in any part of the mouth.

5. Teeth that are getting loose without any reason.

6. Difficulty in swallowing food or moving your tongue around. You may feel as if something has stuck in your throat.

7. Persistent hoarseness of voice or change in voice that does not go away.

8. Dentures that do not fit properly like they used to fit previously or dentures that are getting loose without any obvious reason.

Why Aren't Oral Symptoms Easily Noticed?

You can easily misjudge or ignore oral symptoms because lesions come and go quite often in the oral cavity for different reasons. They look similar to dangerous precancerous lesions and, because they are painless in the beginning, they can easily be missed.

I remember a patient with a thick velvety white patch on the inner lining of his cheek. He would not agree to get a biopsy done because the lesion was painless and was not giving him any problems. Later on, it turned out to be a precancerous lesion. Timely surgery done by an oral surgeon saved this patient's life. You don't have to wait for surgery. Listen to your dentist.

Other Causes of Oral Lesions

One cause of oral lesions can be trauma from the bristles of your toothbrush, which may cause ulceration of gingival tissue. Other causes can be chronic irritation from sharp edges of broken and badly decayed teeth, or from broken old fillings and crowns. That can result in redness and ulceration of surrounding tissues if it keeps irritating tissues slowly over a long time.

In my observations, some patients have caused ulcerations on the inside linings of their cheeks because they were in the habit of cheek biting. You may cause ulceration on your lips if you bite your lips quite often. You can burn your tongue or palate with burning hot pizza or other foods and cause redness. My father used to injure his gums by repeatedly using toothpicks to remove leftover food particles collected between his teeth.

Who is Most Prone to Oral Cancer?

Age itself is a big risk factor. The older you get, the more risk you add. And your family history counts, too.

If you smoke or chew tobacco or beetle nut, you are at high risk for oral cancers. Smoking pipes and cigars practically have the same risk as cigarette smoking. Alcoholism with smoking makes it even worse.

You add another risk factor for cancer on the lips when you spend long hours in the sun.

Nine Tips for Action

1. Get cancer screening done in your dental office for early detection during routine check-ups.

2. Quit your smoking habit and stop chewing beetle nuts or beetle leaves, called paan.

3. Use lip balm or sunscreen and hats or visors to avoid sun damage.

4. Brush your teeth in a proper manner to not to injure the tissues.

5.   Get the sharp edges of your teeth fixed. Restore your broken fillings and crowns.

6.   Follow a healthy lifestyle. Eat balanced foods full of antioxidants. Include all kinds of fresh fruits, vegetables, whole grains, lentils, and legumes.

7.   Add twenty to thirty minutes of walking or aerobic exercise of your choice to your daily routine.

8.   Report any ulcer or canker sore that does not heal within fifteen to twenty days to your dental office, especially if you are forty years or older.

9.   Learn to deal with stress and anxiety with patience if that is the cause for your cheek or lip biting. Take few deep breaths before stressful situations arise.

Now that you have discovered the dangers of tobacco, are you ready to turn to the next chapter to understand that bad breath may be an indicator that something is wrong?

Chapter 13

Toothache Solutions—No Need to Face the Embarrassment of Bad Breath and Related Dental Problems

Do you avoid fun parties or resist meeting people because your breath smells bad? Are you embarrassed to discuss this problem with your friends or with your own doctor or dentist?

After reading this chapter, you will learn why you suffer with this problem and how you can get rid of the bad odor from your mouth so you can meet with your friends without any fear.

Why Does Breath Smell Bad?

Bad breath or foul mouth odor is called halitosis. It is an indicator that either something is wrong in the oral cavity or something is wrong somewhere else in the body, which is called a systemic disorder. The odor is like a wakening call to find out what's happening in the mouth or in the rest of the body.

Halitosis from Oral Cavity

Halitosis can be caused by sulfur-producing bacteria that live and hide in the back part of the tongue and produce a foul smell.

The most obvious cause of bad breath is poor oral hygiene. When teeth are not cleaned properly, they get covered with too much plaque and hard tartar. That makes teeth smell bad.

Gum disease, whether it is initial gingivitis or advanced periodontal disease with red, inflamed, swollen, and bleeding gums, can lead to a strong foul odor from the mouth.

Badly decayed teeth that collect lots of leftover food particles and debris are also responsible for bad breath.

Bad odor from the mouth is also related to eating certain raw foods. Onions and garlic are notorious for halitosis. White radish is another one you can count on.

Smoking cigarettes or chewing tobacco produces a foul odor called smoker's breath. Drinking alcohol, beer, wine, and other alcoholic drinks also add to this unpleasant breath.

Denture wearers face bad mouth odor if dentures are not brushed and cleaned properly every day. People call it denture breath.

Dry mouth may be responsible for halitosis. Dry mouth means there is less flow of saliva. Saliva helps in washing away the leftover food particles and neutralizing the acids produced by bacteria in plaque. If ignored, dry mouth can cause decay in teeth and related pain and discomfort. The leftover food debris and decayed teeth result in foul odor.

Mouth breathing can cause bad breath. Think of a small child who has bad breath when his or her nose is blocked, perhaps from a common cold. Adults who sleep with their mouths open may end up with dry mouth and halitosis.

Halitosis from Systemic Disorder

If oral health is not the causative factor of bad breath, consult your physician to find out if any systemic disease is the cause of this problem.

Halitosis can be associated with certain diseases, like infection in the respiratory tract, sinus infection, or post-nasal drip. Chronic bronchitis can cause foul odor from the mouth. Even persistent constipation can become the cause of bad odor.

Certain medications used commonly for allergy, depression, and anxiety have the side effect of making the mouth dry and thus will result in unpleasant breath.

Ten Tips for Action

1. Brush your tongue once a day with soft toothbrush. Start to brush the tongue from the back very delicately with soft strokes. Use a tongue scraper to remove the soft plaque and decomposed food particles that hide on the back part of the tongue.

2. Consult your dentist for treatment of gum infection before it becomes painful and serious gum disease.

3. Get your decayed teeth fixed with proper fillings before they result in severe pain or loss of teeth.

4. Remove your dentures two to three times a day and brush the dentures, with a special denture brush, just like you would brush your own teeth. That will help to keep the breath fresh. Also, clean your entire mouth by brushing your tongue, palate, and inside of mouth with a soft toothbrush.

5. Rinse your mouth with water after every meal to remove the leftover food particles. Use antibacterial mouthwash once a day.

6. Drink plenty of water to keep your mouth moist.

7. Chew sugarless gum to increase flow of saliva for dry mouth.

8.   Inform your physician or dentist about the problem, and replace or change medications if they are causing dry mouth and are not tolerable.

9.   Freshen your breath with healthy, baked fennel seeds and cardamom pods like people do in India. Chew on these after meals for fresh breath and good digestion.

10.   Practice good oral hygiene to keep plaque under control. Brush at least twice a day and floss once a day.

Now that you know the primary cause of bad breath, get ready to discover in the next chapter how certain medications can cause oral problems for you.

Chapter 14

Toothache Solutions—Find Out Which Oral Lesions Are the Side Effects of Medications

Are you concerned about bitter taste and sore spots in your mouth? Are you are worried about swollen gums that are overgrowing your teeth? Maybe you are wondering why your child's baby teeth are a brownish color?

In this chapter, you will find out how certain medications you take for pain, allergy, depression, and the common cold can cause oral lesions and other problems. You may want to replace them or let go of them.

Some Commonly Used Medicines That Change Taste

- Antibiotics
- Allergy medications
- Drugs used for fungal infections
- Asthma medications
- High blood pressure medications
- Drugs taken for cancer

A new antibiotic named Clarithromycin is especially known for causing a strange metallic taste. Lots of other medicines cause bitter to salty tastes. The good news is, as soon as you stop the medicines, the bad taste disappears.

What Makes Gums Overgrown?

A few medications, such as dilantin sodium, can cause overgrowth of gum tissue called gingival hyperplasia. The gum tissue becomes so swollen that it starts to grow over the teeth. This medication is given to patients with seizure disorder, also known as epilepsy. I remember seeing one patient whose teeth got almost completely covered with overgrowth of swollen gums because of long-term use of this drug. Swollen gum tissues are an ideal place to collect plaque. If plaque is not removed on a regular basis, it can result in bleeding gums, cavities, and tooth pain.

Why Do Teeth Get Discolored?

Some medicines are responsible for discolored teeth. The antibiotic tetracycline is well known to cause discoloration of baby teeth if given to pregnant mothers because baby teeth are still in the developmental stage in the jaws during pregnancy. However, once the teeth are fully formed, tetracycline does not cause any discoloration.

The other drug called chlorhexidine is a good antiseptic or disinfectant oral rinse. But the biggest disadvantage is that it can cause really bad stains on your teeth. When I used this oral rinse, my teeth turned dark brown in color within one week, so I had to stop using it.

Which Medicines Cause Dry Mouth?

A common side effect of many medicines is reducing saliva in the mouth that leads to dry mouth. Saliva keeps the mouth moist and washes away leftover food particles. With less saliva, you become more prone to cavities, gingivitis, and pain. A few examples of these include medications used for:

- Allergy
- Depression
- Alzheimer's and Parkinson's
- Chemotherapy in cancer patients
- Anxiety
- High blood pressure
- Sleeping disorders
- Colds, such as sweet cough syrups given to small children

Some Miscellaneous Oral Lesions

Oral manifestations are seen with methamphetamine abuse. It causes reduction in salivary flow, leading to dry mouth. A rapidly progressing form of dental caries called meth mouth has been seen. With this drug abuse, people have a tendency for grinding and clenching teeth. These forces can break old fillings and fracture the teeth and make them sensitive to hot and cold.

Some antibiotics, or inhalers used for asthma, can cause a fungal infection called candidiasis or thrush if used for a longer period of time. This causes whitish or yellow flecks or plaques with a smooth and slightly raised appearance. These lesions can happen anywhere on the mucosal lining of the mouth and cause an uncomfortable feeling. The surfaces of these lesions can be removed easily, but they leave a reddish base underneath that may bleed.

Eight Tips for Action

1. Inform your dentist about all the medications you are taking.

2. Keep your teeth clean and free of plaque if you have enlarged and swollen gums. By keeping teeth clean, this condition may reverse itself.

3. Check with your dentist about gum surgery. It may be needed in severe cases of gum enlargement.

4. Avoid taking tetracycline or replace it with other antibiotics if you are pregnant.

5. Drink a lot of water to keep your mouth moist to prevent dry mouth. Chewing sugarless gum increases the flow of saliva.

6. Ask your physician or dentist to change or replace medications if side effects are too irritating or painful.

7. Avoid spicy, sour, and hot foods if you have ulcers or sore spots in your mouth.

8. Get your teeth professionally cleaned and polished if your teeth are brownish from chlorhexidine oral rinse.

Now that you are aware of how medical conditions and certain medications affect your oral health, look into the final chapter of this book to see how your mouth and your body are interconnected.

Chapter 15

Toothache Solutions—Find Out Which Dental Problems Are a Result of Mouth-Body Connection

Do you wonder why you have an occasional burning sensation and dryness in your mouth? Do you worry about loose teeth without any obvious reasons? Maybe looking at those grayish- white patches on your tongue surprises you?

In this chapter, you will find out which of your medical problems give these signals in the mouth because of the mouth-body connection. And your dentist may be the first person to make the diagnosis.

What is Mouth-Body Connection?

Ancient texts point out that in old times, physicians used to examine a patient's mouth and tongue very carefully to make the diagnosis for problems happening in the rest of the body. No fancy tests were available at that time. They believed in what we call today the mouth-body connection, and they looked in the mouth as a mirror of the whole body.

Connection Between Gum Disease and Heart Disease?

Scientists have discovered that healthy gums are important for a healthy heart. Poor oral health can increase your chances of developing cardiovascular disease. If you are suffering with periodontal disease, you are at high risk for heart problems and stroke.

Connection Between Oral Health and Hormonal Changes?

Women are more prone to gum disease or periodontal disease whenever hormonal change happens—at puberty, pregnancy, and menopause. Healthy teeth and gums are important for a healthy baby if you are pregnant. You may deliver a premature baby or your baby may be below the normal weight if you have been suffering with periodontal disease during pregnancy.

Postmenopausal women may feel that their mouths and lips are very dry. The tongue may get dry and red, too. My mother always complains that hot and spicy food hurts her because she has extremely dry lips with deep fissures and cracked skin at the corners of her mouth that extends onto the adjacent skin. This is another postmenopausal symptom that affects oral health. An occasional burning sensation in the mouth is another symptom.

Does Diabetes Connect with Mouth?

With diabetes, you have a higher level of glucose in saliva, which can make you more prone to get cavities in your teeth.

If your diabetes is not under control, you are likely to face recurrent oral infections because of lowered resistance to infections. You will be more susceptible to inflamed, swollen, and bleeding gums. If you ignore these signs, it can turn to an advanced stage of periodontal disease, with eventual loss of bone and tissues that support your teeth.

One side effect of diabetes is thirst caused from a dry mouth. You may also feel an occasional burning sensation in your mouth. Your wound healing may be delayed. A foul odor may come from your mouth.

You may not be aware that you are suffering with uncontrolled diabetes. With all oral symptoms, your dentist may be the first person to make the diagnosis.

Profuse Gum Bleeding

Unexplained profuse bleeding from gums indicates that you may be suffering with extreme deficiency of vitamin C. Do you remember scurvy or pellagra? Fortunately, we don't have these diseases in the United States. But it is commonly seen in underprivileged countries where people are extremely malnourished.

Hemophilia, a blood disorder, is sometimes diagnosed by dentists because of incidental bleeding during dental work.

Loose Teeth

If you wonder why your teeth get loose with no obvious reason, it could be a signal that you may have osteoporosis. With osteoporosis, people have low bone density and the bones gradually become fragile. The thinning of bones can affect the jawbones, which support the teeth. You may not be aware of you have osteoporosis, and your dentist might be the first person to make the diagnosis.

Grayish Patches Inside the Mouth

If you see white-grayish patches on your tongue or inside the cheeks, it indicates thrush or a yeast infection called oral candidiasis. It happens when you've suffered with chronic sickness that has lowered your resistance to infections.

You see this oral candidiasis in little babies, also, if they get exposed to infections, as their immune systems are not fully developed yet.

Dry Mouth and Lips

Certain diseases like Sjorgen's Syndrome are known for making the mouth dry because of reduction in salivary flow. This can also cause dry lips and cracks or fissures in the corners of your mouth that extend onto the adjacent skin.

Systemic chemotherapy and radiotherapy for treatment of cancers in or around head and neck area will decrease the salivary flow and cause dry mouth and lips. That happens as salivary glands that produce saliva get exposed to radiation.

Why Do Hot and Cold Foods Hurt My Teeth?

You may have thinning of enamel from gastroesophageal reflux disease, called GERD for short. In this disorder, acid from the stomach comes into the mouth. The extended cumulative exposure of tooth enamel to this acidic mixture results in eroding the hard layer of enamel, making small cavities called erosion cavities. The erosion extends through the enamel into the dentin and yields a small, smooth, and glossy surface. That makes your teeth sensitive to hot, cold, sour, and sweet stuff. Exposed dentin is softer than enamel and thus is more prone to caries, also.

I remember a patient who was unable to understand why his teeth hurt all the time with hot and cold foods when he had a very clean mouth and no decayed teeth. After taking his medical history and looking at the thinning of enamel on his teeth, I pointed out that it was related to gastroesophageal reflux. This patient was not aware that he suffered with GERD. After being referred to his physician, he got proper treatment.

Similar oral complications happen from an eating disorder called bulimia nervosa because of binge eating and self-induced vomiting.

Why Do I Get Recurrent Canker Sores?

Most common and painful sore spots in the mouth are known as aphthous ulcers, or canker sores. They can happen anywhere on the inner lining of cheeks, lips, soft palate, or floor of mouth. They are so painful that they can interfere with your normal eating, swallowing, and talking. Physical and emotional stress may cause it. Your family history could be one of the causes. Or it could be related to nutritional deficiencies, such as a vitamin B complex deficiency.

Nine Tips for Action

1. Make regular visits to your dental office to discover these problems at their earliest stages. You can avoid many problems with early detection.

2. Take calcium regularly to prevent oste-oporosis and to keep bones strong, including jawbones.

3. Include vitamin D supplement in your diet, as it helps to absorb calcium in the body.

4. Drink lots of water for a dry mouth. Chewing sugarless gum increases the flow of saliva.

5. Consult with your physician for treatment of GERD and diabetes.

6. Keep your gums healthy for a healthy heart. Eat balanced food and plenty of fruits from the citrus family.

7. For women, keep your gums in good health for healthy babies. Practice good oral hygiene at home, and have routine check-ups in your dental office.

8. Avoid sour, spicy, and hot food for an extremely dry mouth, tongue, cracked lips, and canker sores.

9. Avoid foods with sharp edges that can cause physical trauma to painful lesions of canker sores.

MISCELLANEOUS

COMMONLY USED DENTAL TERMS

ADA: American Dental Association

Bruxism: grinding of teeth or clenching of teeth

Calculus: hard deposits on teeth

Caries: medical term for decay in teeth

Cavity: a hole in the teeth

Cusp: a projection on chewing surfaces of back teeth

Diastema: spacing between teeth

Dentin: inner layer of tooth structure, underneath the hard layer of enamel

Dentures: removable artificial teeth to replace missing natural teeth

Enamel: hard mineralized layer on teeth that covers only crown of tooth

Fixed crown: cap placed on damaged tooth, which is cemented on the tooth to stay there permanently

Full denture: artificial replacement of all upper and lower teeth

Gingiva: medical term for gums

Gingivitis: inflammation of gums

Gingival hyperplasia: overgrowth of gum tissue

Halitosis: bad odor from mouth

Impacted tooth: tooth sitting inside the jaw that never erupts in mouth

Implants: artificial teeth with metal posts, done surgically

Incisors: four upper and four lower front teeth

Malocclusion: when teeth or jaws are not in normal alignment

Molars: main chewing teeth toward back of mouth

Mouth guard: a custom-made device worn over the teeth to protect them

Non-vital tooth: a tooth whose nerve died from trauma or decay

Occlusal surface: chewing surface of molars and premolars

Occlusion: when teeth and jaws are in normal alignment

Partial denture: artificial teeth to replace one or more teeth

Periodontitis: inflammation of gums and supporting structures

Pits: small grooves on occlusal surface of molars and premolars

Plaque: soft, sticky film of bacteria on teeth

Premolar: teeth in front of molars, also called bicuspids

Prophylaxis: routine cleaning and polishing in dental office

Proximal cavity: cavity on that surface of tooth that is toward adjacent tooth

Radiographs: X-rays

Saliva: clear lubricating fluid in the mouth

Scaling and root planing: deep cleaning to remove hard tartar from teeth; above and below the gum line and root surfaces are made smooth

Tartar: hard deposits on teeth, also called calculus

Temporomandibular joint: name of the joint where lower jaw connects with upper jaw in front of ears

Thrush: a fungal infection in mouth

Trauma: injury caused by forceful brushing, extremely hot foods, or external blow to the face

Trismus: restricted opening of mouth

Unilateral mastication: eating food only on one side of mouth

Veneer: thin, custom-made shell of tooth-colored material placed on the tooth surface

Xerostomia: dryness of mouth

DENTAL SPECIALISTS

Cosmetic dentist: a dentist who has special training in using the latest techniques to reshape and recontour the teeth to improve a patient's appearance

Endodontist: a dentist who specializes in root-canal treatment and associated work

Pedodontist: a dentist who specializes in taking care of children until the age of twelve years

Prosthodontist: a dentist who specializes in replacing missing teeth

Oral and maxillofacial surgeon: a dentist who specializes in surgical treatments around mouth and jaws, including surgical removal of impacted wisdom teeth

Orthodontist: a dentist who specializes in correcting abnormal bite when teeth or jaws are not in normal alignment

CONTACT INFORMATION

You can contact us at

www.toothachesolutions.com

Visit us on.....

www.toothachesolutions.com/facebook/

ACKNOWLEDGMENTS

My sincere thanks goes to my husband, Dr. Devinder Tandon, MD, FCCP, for his never-ending support and confidence for my work, and his contribution for systemic diseases affecting oral health, and their mouth body connection with numerous tips. Devinder Tandon is a former chief of medicine and director of respiratory therapy department of Simi Adventist Hospital California.

My heartfelt thanks goes to my daughter Geetika, a co writer for NBC's comedy show "Outsourced", for her help in editing the book.

I am extremely grateful to Dr. Harbans Bhatia DDS, my mentor and my teacher for reading the whole manuscript and giving his wise opinion for every chapter in this book. He practiced dentistry in Los Angeles, California for more than 35 years.

My warmest thanks go to all my children including Geetika and Manish and their spouses Steven and Poonam for their help and continuous encouragement in the completion of this book.

My special thanks go to my favorite book coach and editor Judy Cullins for making my dream into reality. Without her help I couldn't have put book into this great shape. Judy has authored 13 books including "Write your eBook or Other Short Book Fast".

I must mention thanks to my grandchildren Devin, Sofia and Dylan who always brush their teeth before they go to bed and never miss their routine dental appointments to their pedodontist's office.

Many thanks to my friends Sarita and Shamim who have been my biggest encouragement to finish this book.

Last but not the least thanks I want to say is to Vaneet Khanna, Tarun Viz and Jessica Danai, who were always there for me whenever I had panic attacks with my computer.

Frequently Asked Questions
About Dental Health

FREQUENTLY ASKED QUESTIONS

Q. If I brush and floss every day at home, is it still important for me to have a prophylaxis (a routine cleaning by a dentist or dental hygienist)?

A. It's great that you are doing your share of keeping your teeth clean. However, you still need a dentist or dental hygienist to remove the calculus and stains and to polish your teeth, as you cannot remove the hard tartar or calculus with brushing and flossing at home. In addition, the dentist will also look for early signs of cavities or any other dental problems.

Q. Is my diet important for healthy teeth?

A. Certainly, it is important just like it is important for the health of any organs in the body.

Q. What is a balanced diet? Why is breakfast the most important meal of the day?

A. A well-balanced diet consists of enough varieties of food to give you the essential proteins and minerals necessary for normal growth and maintenance of health. The most important meal of the day is breakfast. It gives you energy for the whole day's work. Not eating breakfast and having a large evening meal would be like going on a 1000-mile trip and adding fuel after you get there.

Q. Does excessive eating of sweets cause gum disease?

A. Excessive eating of sweets does not in itself cause gum disease. However, it does weaken the body's defenses, making it easier for disease to attack gums.

Q. How does eating sweets affect the health of my mouth?

A. Sugars are turned into acids by the bacteria in the mouth. Acids attack the enamel on the teeth. By repeated acid attack, the protective coating of enamel dissolves, resulting in cavities on teeth. It must be emphasized that in a clean mouth, free of plaque and sugar, cannot damage the teeth.

Q. Are X-Rays necessary to diagnose gum disease?

A. No, not always. Early gum disease is best diagnosed by either the presence of bleeding gums or the formation of calculus on the necks of teeth. No damage is visible in X-rays at the beginning stage. In advanced gum disease, called pyorrhea or periodontal disease, X-rays definitely help to determine the amount of damage done to underlying bone and supporting structures.

Q. What are gum boils?

A. Gum boils are usually caused by badly decayed and infected teeth or by advanced pyorrhea. They can be cured, but it is best to prevent them before they happen.

Q. Are canker sores and mouth ulcers caused by gum disease?

A. No, they are not. They are produced by a virus in the tissues. When the body's resistance is lowered, the virus becomes active and creates the typical lesion.

Q. What is the reason for space between the front teeth?

A. The space between teeth is called diastema. This space can occur in adults with severe gum disease when teeth get loose and start shifting. In children, it is often produced by the habit of tongue thrusting.

Q. Why do I get food impactions between some of my teeth?

A. If food is forced between the teeth during eating, it is most likely due to an improper match of upper and lower teeth. It can also happen in the presence of proximal cavities, which are formed between two adjoining teeth.

Q. My gums used to bleed during brushing and sometimes while eating. Now the bleeding has subsided, and I think that my mouth is healthy. How can I be sure?

A. It is possible that either your mouth has become healthy or the disease has advanced to the next stage, where the infection is too deep to produce gingival bleeding. It is best to check with your dentist, who will use a periodontal probe to check the pocket depth to rule out periodontal disease. Healthy gums have a one-millimeter or less crevice depth; three millimeters or more denotes gum disease.

TESTIMONIALS

Praise from happy readers:

This is a must-read book for everyone looking for a small, practical guide to explore and understand toothache problems and their remedies to enjoy pain-free teeth. This can be a great reference guide for every household.

Chand Khanna, MD, FCCP

Director of Pulmonary Department

Former Chief of Staff at Henry Mayo Hospital, Valencia, CA.

It's a great book, easy to read, and full of practical information about how to keep and maintain your original adult teeth well into your 80s and 90s. A must-read for anyone and everyone who savors their teeth and love of food.

Parvesh Kumar, MD

Associate Director of Clinical Research, KU Cancer Center

University of Kansas Medical Center

I particularly enjoy the way Dr. Tandon clearly explains the dental problems, what caused them, how one problem leads to another problem, and how to prevent the problems (or at least halt the damage) to begin with. It is obvious that her goal is to keep our teeth healthy and thus keep our whole mind and body healthy also.

Rebecca Lizardi

12th grade school teacher

I highly admire Dr. Usha Tandon's integrity, her passion, and her tremendous efforts to bring forth this handbook of dental queries to help relieve patients' anxiety somewhat when they are in a dental chair. Kudos to her for thinking about something so useful and prevention-oriented in the everyday dental world.

Vanna Master, DDS

General dentist in Thousand Oaks, CA

This little book, packed with a wealth of knowledge, is an excellent home health resource for a wide variety of dental problems. It can make a remarkable difference

in everyone's life at this time when it is most needed.

Feri Afshar, DDS, MS

Pedodontist from Simi Valley, CA

ABOUT THE AUTHOR

Dr. Usha Tandon graduated from dental school in India and stayed on as teaching staff member of the dental school for some time. She worked in public health dental clinics in Kentucky. She practiced general dentistry in Los Angeles, California, for more than sixteen years.

In her practice, Usha spent a great deal of time educating patients not only about their dental health, but also about their physical and mental well-being.

Every time she visits India, she distributes toothbrushes to children in orphanages, teaches them the proper method of brushing, and talks to them about the benefits of taking good care of their dental health from a young age.